REBOUNDING
FOR
HEALTH

MARGARET HAWKINS

THE REBOUNDER CENTRE
Leicester

First Edition, 1993, Rebounding for Health & Fitness
published by Thorsons, an imprint of HarperCollins*Publishers*

Reprinted, 1996, Rebounding for Health

published by M & P Hawkins
THE REBOUNDER CENTRE
51 Nevanthon Road
Leicester LE3 6DR

© Margaret Hawkins 1993

Margaret Hawkins asserts the moral right to
be identified as the author of the work

A catalogue record for this book is
available from the British Library

ISBN 0 9520780 1 5

Illustrations by Andrea Norton

Printed in Great Britain
by Norwood Press, Anstey, Leicester.

Also by Margaret Hawkins:

in conjuction with Melissa Tunaley –
REBOUND AEROBICS

Video – *CARDIO BOUNCE PLUS*
The Total Vitality Plan for Rebounders

'Those who think they have not time for bodily exercise will sooner or later have to find time for illness.'

EDWARD STANLEY, EARL OF DERBY
'The Conduct of Life' –
an address at Liverpool College, December 1873

For over five years we have been working mainly with people who are ill or old. But as time has gone on we have realised more and more that there is a great need for an exercise that is very easy and very quick and that is suitable for all, so that young and old, fit and unfit, and even the lazy can keep themselves in a state of wellness that will help them cope with life.

THIS IS IT!

We have heard from people with a wide variety of illnesses and here is a list of the things that rebounding has helped:

Ageing

Allergies

Arthritis – rheumatoid and osteo-

Asthma

Back Pain

Blood Pressure

Catarrh

Cholesterol and Circulation

Colds, Influenza and Sore Throats

Constipation

Depression

Diabetes

General Health

Hyperactivity

Migraine

Multiple Sclerosis

Myalgic Encephalomyelitis – ME

Osteoporosis

Parkinson's Disease

Premenstrual Tension

Skin, Hair and Nails

Sleeping Problems

Slimming

Sports Injuries

Stress and Tension

Strokes

Varicose Veins

Acknowledgements

I would like to acknowledge the support and enthusiasm of Dr Neuburg and Dr Sheehan and also to thank John and Philippa Turville for their help and support through the last five years.

Many thanks to the many hundreds of people who not only took us seriously and tried rebounding, but also took the trouble to contact us and tell us what has happened to them. Without them we could not have gained much of the knowledge to write this book and it's thanks to their help and information that we have now been able to help many thousands of others whose lives have been altered by rebounding.

Thanks to our daughter, Melissa, who now works with us. Her speciality is rebound aerobics. My most loving thanks to Peter, my husband, for his patience and for having the courage to give up his lifetime profession as an insurance broker when he was near retirement to go out with me to spread the word and help me establish the Rebounder Centre in Leicester. There we work with everyone from the young and fit to the older, some up to 90 odd years old, and the ill. And thanks to Peter not least for all his hard work in the preparation and typing of this book.

I would like to thank Sarah Sutton (our editor) for her patience and kindness in helping us to bring this book to press.

Contents

Preface

For 14 years I had suffered from rheumatoid arthritis and also had a multi-allergy disease which meant that I was allergic to some 90 different foods and chemicals, including dairy produce, grains, most fish, petrol, diesel oil, gas, smoke, and also sunshine. I seemed to live on soya beans and fruit and life was very difficult. In fact I had a breakdown of the immune system. I was having difficulty in walking, my hands and arms were just a mass of pain. Some days I had a job even to cut up my food, and holding a cup was a two-handed job. I was only in my fifties but felt more like 80. Just to get a meal for my family was a mammoth task and the nights seemed to go on for ever as I was in too much pain to sleep.

Six years ago, just after I had given up my part-time work, I read that in America geriatrics with arthritis were being treated on rebounders. **I wanted one**. I was willing to try anything, but although I asked doctors, physiotherapists and, in fact, anyone who would listen, nobody seemed to have heard the word 'rebounder'. We knew that it looked like a little round trampoline, but that was all. Then, in 1988, our younger daughter and her husband came in with a very large box. They were obviously very excited. 'We've got you one, mum,' they said, and unpacked a little trampoline. I got onto it very carefully and tried to bounce. I felt terrified; it was springy and bouncy and I felt unsafe. If that was a rebounder, I knew that I could not use one.

Three weeks later Peter, my husband, and I went on holiday and there in the leisure complex was a rebounder. It was quite different from a trampoline. It was firm and solid with very little bounce.

I stepped onto it *very* carefully and bounced *very gently* for about 30 seconds. Almost immediately my hands started to tingle. I could feel things happening. The only thing I knew about using a rebounder was that you have to use it frequently, so while I was there I used it three times a day. By the end of that week I felt very different. The pain in my arms had lifted. Until then I had been in such terrible pain that I used to be frightened of going out into a crowd in case someone should knock me. Now I felt taller, fitter and also had a sense of well-being and energy – a feeling that I had not had for many years. This was incredible and although I could only bounce for 30 seconds at a time, I liked it. It made me feel good, as though my body was coming back to life. I wanted to smile.

Within about four days of getting back home my pain had come back. My feeling of energy and well-being had gone. I felt smaller, older and back to normal. I felt terribly depressed, almost worse than before. I had suddenly felt better and had had that wonderful feeling of energy and well-being, and then just as suddenly it had gone.

Shortly after this I managed to get a rebounder of my own and started to use it very gently. After about four days my pain eased and I got back my feeling of well-being and energy. It was marvellous and it was obvious that this was what the rebounder was doing. This was it – IT WORKS!

Suddenly things started to happen; it was as if someone else had taken charge. We found a survey on rebounders telling us that there was only one that was completely safe. More important we found out where to get one. We also learned what happens in your body when you bounce, and the fact that in a few minutes each day it could help people – young, old, fit or in fact very ill – to get fitter and healthier.

People with arthritis, ME, Parkinson's disease, MS, asthma, diabetes, varicose veins and many other illnesses are benefiting. Rebounding is a way that everyone can use to get gradually fitter, healthier and happier. Most hospitals are using them for physiotherapy and as part of rehabilitation after heart surgery. It is also a wonderful way to get slimmer, fitter and healthier in only minutes a day in your own home. Some people have lost three to four stone (42 to 56 pounds) by rebounding for two or three minutes, two or three times a day.

I have regained my strength and health, reduced my pain and regained the feeling that life is worth living again; I hope that reading this book will help you to do the same. As you will realise from the following chapters, exercise is an amazing thing and can improve the quality of life enormously, and rebound exercise is easy and painless. It does not impose the skeletal shock on one's body usually associated with exercise, but will keep you fit or get you fitter easily, quickly, and with a minimum of effort.

Introduction: Why Rebound?

Rebounding works like any other exercise, so why rebound when you could jog, skip, cycle, swim or any other form of vigorous physical activity?

First let me ask you a question: Do you do any of these things for at least 30 to 40 minutes three times a week? If not, why not? Time is a big problem for many people. There are also many who simply do not like normal exercise and those who are just not well enough to cope with it. How would you like an execise that takes only a few minutes a day, and that is so easy that almost everyone can do it? Rebounding is that exercise. We know of many 90-year-olds who rebound daily. There is no skeletal shock and it's fun.

Dr Alexander Leaf MD in his book *Youth in Old Age* points out that the difference between our bodies and, say, a car is that the car can only deteriorate with age, whereas our bodies can improve with usage provided we are in good health and the activity is not too violent. As you rebound you are doing what every form of exercise does and using gravity – defeating it for short periods of time and being subjected to an apparently higher level of it in between. This gently stresses all the muscles in the body simultaneously and with a minimum of effort. Ten minutes on a rebounder will give you the same benefits as a 30-minute jog but without the skeletal shock. This means that many who could not normally exercise can take advantage of the gentleness of rebounding and gain all the benefits usually associated with exercise, without placing undue stress on an already hampered body.

Almost everyone could be fitter by spending only minutes a day on a rebounder, and we can all find a few minutes however busy we are. You can rebound in your own home and you do not need any special clothing or footwear: unless you are doing a fairly vigorous and extensive workout you are best rebounding in bare feet, and you do not need to shower afterwards. You can even watch television while you exercise. It is, however, most important to use the correct equipment in the right way and we shall go into this in depth later in the book.

Why rebound instead of some other form of exercise? In short, IT'S QUICK, IT'S EASY, IT'S CONVEN-IENT, IT'S FUN AND IT WORKS.

How Did Rebounding Start?

The first documented information about the health aspects of rebounding came from ex-professional wrestler Albert Carter in a book called *The Miracle of Rebound Exercise*. Albert and his family were all proficient on the trampoline. One day his daughter announced that she had been arm wrestling with the boys and had won. His son started wrestling and Albert realised that he was stronger, fitter, quicker and better balanced than his opponents. At this time Albert was 36 and still able to do over 100 single-arm push-ups and had a resting pulse of 39 beats per minute. None of them did any training other than trampolining, so he decided to research it, only to find that there was no mention of it in any of the exercise books.

Albert knew that any form of training or strengthening exercise needs some form of opposition, since without opposition no strength is needed and no effort is used, so the training effect is nil.

One night when he was travelling by air across the United States he suddenly realised that the one thing that all exercise has in common is that to a greater or lesser extent it involves defeating gravity. Following on from this thought he realised that trampolining harnesses three powerful forces – gravity, acceleration and deceleration. Most of you will have experienced that feeling in an aircraft when it quickly accelerates and you are forced back into your seat and cannot move. It is as if gravity has increased and you are not strong enough to overcome it.

Although your body does not seem to recognise the difference between gravity and acceleration, it does automatically strengthen itself to cope with the worst conditions that it repeatedly encounters. Consequently when you are putting your body under an apparent one and a half times normal gravity ($1\frac{1}{2}$G) it will strengthen itself to a level to cope adequately with this condition. As a result the body gradually becomes stronger in each cell and as a consequence of that all the muscles and organs become stronger. What rebounding does is to harness and use the force of gravity effectively.

At the top of the bounce your body becomes completely weightless and this stimulates the lymphatic flow. This gravity/non-gravity repetition occurs about 100 times each minute, so the body quickly strengthens a little. The lymphatic circulation also improves to bring about greater efficiency in the clearing of waste matter in the body and in the effectiveness of the immune system.

The next step was the development of a trampoline that was lower off the ground and had less bounce than a traditional trampoline, to avoid the dangers normally associated with trampolining, and rebounding had arrived.

The American space agency, NASA, made a study of the training effect of trampolining and found that use of a trampoline below the level where you reach a jump of 4G (four times normal gravity) is up to 68 per cent more oxygen efficient than other forms of exercise. That means that you can exercise quite strenuously for your condition without feeling out of breath, but still gain the same benefit as you would from much more strenuous exercise on a hard surface. A rebounder should restrict the level to which you can bounce to below 4G and, in fact, a good rebounder will keep you below 3½G to be on the safe side.

NASA also found that there is much less likelihood of taking cells, particularly those in the ankles, knees and lower back, above their cell rupture level and consequently causing pain. When they measured the stress on the ankles, the small of the back and the forehead, NASA found that on a hard surface the stress level was twice as much at the ankle as at the forehead or small of the back, whereas on a trampoline the stress level was almost the same. This helps to explain how rebounding avoids the shinsplint and knee problems that arise from traditional forms of exercise.

The NASA research also showed that rebounding helped restore the bone mass that astronauts had lost in space, and subsequent medical trials in the USA have shown that it can stop osteoporosis (brittleness of the bones) getting any worse. It may, in fact, reverse the deterioration caused by osteoporosis, but this has not yet been medically accepted. As one woman in four will develop osteoporosis, and as osteoporosis-related accidents can be fatal, arresting the deterioration is clearly important.

Rebounding Now

Rebounders are now successfully being used in the USA to treat people with arthritis and also people with mental disorders. Many physiotherapy departments are using rebounders as part of their rehabilitation programmes. They are used to treat a wide variety of conditions, including sports injuries and non-sports conditions, such as bad backs, shinsplints, and as part of the therapy after heart surgery. Why not start it first and avoid the heart surgery!

Chapter 1

Why Should I Exercise?

Is good health merely the absence of disease or is it something more? You may remember a time when you wanted to run or leap about for the sheer joy of it – with a little encouragement you felt as if you could make the world go round the other way. You can feel like that again, whatever your age. For most of us the way to real health is entirely within our grasp.

Our bodies were designed to be active – to walk and run and hunt on foot – and although our lives have changed greatly our bodies have not. It may be very convenient to sit in a car but it is hardly the exercise that we need to keep ourselves fit and healthy. It is similarly convenient not to have to leave our chairs to change channels on the television and to leave the washing in the washing-machine to wash itself while the dishes are in the dishwasher being washed up. Great! But daily physical activity is necessary to maintain a healthy body and resistance to disease.

Recent research studies have found that gentle exercise is accompanied by a surge of endorphins, which are the body's potent painkillers, and other naturally occurring chemicals such as serotonin, a natural tranquilliser that gives rise to feelings of calmness and serenity. Many have found that a very gentle form of exercise will help them to sleep better. A stimulation of the production of serotonin will help to reduce the stress of modern life, and stress is, of course, probably one of the most lethal parts of our present way of existence.

Many who have started a programme of physical fitness will tell you that they have found their mental capacities improving along with their physical fitness. Concentration, will-power and the ability to keep going even during extreme fatigue are usually all strengthened by sensible aerobic exercise. The feeling of well-being which the right amount of physical exercise creates carries through into our mental outlook and enables many to widen their horizons and take a much less limited view of their own capabilities. When we feel fit, the grass is greener, the sky is bluer and life becomes a great adventure again.

The Lymphatic System

The average person carries round in their body between four and six pounds (one and three-quarters and two and three-quarters kilos) of toxins and other waste, which has a detrimental effect on both physical and mental health. The body's mechanism for clearing away these toxins and wastes is the lymphatic system.

We have about eight pints of blood in our bodies and a pump to pump the blood round – the heart. We have about 24 pints of lymph as well, three times as much, but there is apparently no pump to circulate it. In fact the lymph is circulated by a system of one-way valves, stimulated by exercise. Lymph fluid carries the rubbish our bodies accumulate through the lymph nodes where the impurities and dead cells are filtered out. The nodes are also the place in which antibodies fight infection and toxins are cleared. In this way the lymphatic system works to clear toxicity and excess mucus and is an important carrier of the immune cells, which help prevent disease, degeneration and aging. An efficient lymphatic system improves your health and gives you a feeling of well-being and energy. It can banish joint pain and help regenerate the body, improving the skin, hair and nails, and strengthening the circulation and cardiovascular system.

Our bodies have no other way of removing toxins and

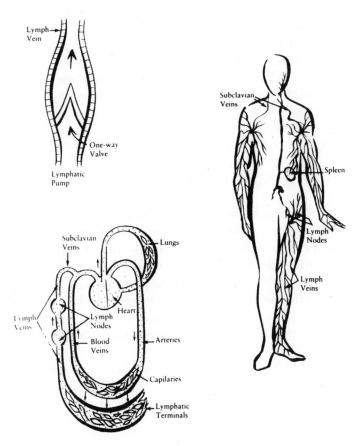

waste from our tissues and cells. Without the waste-eliminating functions of the lymphatic system we would die in about a day. Lack of exercise means a sluggish lymphatic system and consequent poor health.

In order to be effective, most forms of exercise need doing for 30 to 40 minutes at least three times a week. After 48 hours the body starts to lose the stimulation that aerobic exercise gives and without further effort allows the lymphatic circulation to become less vigorous, with the inevitable result that the waste is not moved away and the toxins are allowed to remain.

The easiest way to improve lymphatic circulation is rebounding. The frequent gravity/no gravity repetition that it creates will cause the necessary stimulation with a low physical effort on your part. Rebounding provides the pump to get the lymph moving around again, clearing the way to better health.

Other Benefits of Exercise

A regular programme of aerobic exercise increases energy levels because it changes the body's metabolism. The activity of the mitochondria in the cells is increased to create more ATP (adenosine triphosphate), and ATP is what your body uses when it needs energy to perform some function. Long-term aerobic exercise not only burns fat but also changes the body's capacity to convert fat into energy, and you will therefore burn up fat more effectively even while you are resting.

We have found that most people who are genuinely overweight lose weight steadily if they rebound for two or three minutes three times or more a day. The more frequently you can exercise the better, and the quicker you will start to move that excess weight.

While researching into age and health Dr Alexander Leaf found that in parts of the world where survival to 100 years of age is commonplace people do not appear to have the diseases which are usually all too common in old age in the rest of the world, such as arthritis and heart complaints. Dr Leaf discovered that the common ground for these centogenarians was that they all lived in areas where if you go anywhere you walk and everyone, including them, has to do a good day's physical work for them all to survive. Using modern techniques he studied their heart and lung functions, and found that many did in fact have cardiovascular diseases and arthritis, but they did not display nor were they aware of any of the symptoms.

With any aerobic exercise the heart and lungs are used to a higher capacity and, with the removal of a greater quantity of the waste matter and cholesterol that are in and around the veins and arteries, the heart starts to work with greater efficiency and circulation improves. Many have noticed that their body keeps warmer, as the thermogenic process is able to operate more efficiently with a better supply of fresh blood containing the right amount of oxygen to enable the 'burning' process to work at a higher level.

You may feel that exercising will put you under even more pressure, as you would need to make space in your already busy life for exercise and find the energy to do it. But exercise will increase your capacity for work or any other activity. You will be less likely to be depressed, more likely to be in better shape and have greater stamina, your outlook will become more positive and the world will look a better place. Rebounding is an easy and effective way to achieve these benefits.

Chapter 2

How Rebounding Can Improve Health

I have no medical qualification. I started rebounding to help myself – I was crippled and now I am well. My arthritis has not gone but I can and do live a very busy life. My allergies, all 93 of them, have gone!

In the last six years we have helped many thousands of people to improve the quality of their lives. There is much medical information backing up the results of rebounding, and although its effects are not accepted by all of the medical profession, we are finding that more and more doctors are contacting us saying that their patients are improving greatly since they started to bounce and asked for further information.

We do not, however, claim that rebounding will cure anything. In this chapter we document our own experience and that of others.

Allergies

I had over 90 allergies when I started rebounding. Some were food allergies, others were petrol and diesel fumes, perfume and sunlight. The allergy doctor that I had been visiting said that he thought the stimulation of the lymphatic system caused by rebounding would in the long term probably cure my allergy problem, and in the event, for me, it did. Others have also found that allergies have reduced or gone altogether.

The stimulation of the lymphatic circulation will certainly make the immune system more efficient, although strengthening the immune system to the point of clearing allergies is not quick. It took me about 18 months to clear mine, but whilst you are doing this your body will be getting fitter and healthier.

Arthritis

It was my rheumatoid arthritis that started me rebounding. At Elks Hospital in Idaho, USA, Dr Kenneth Smith, head of the Department of Rehabilitation, did extensive tests involving 2,300 patients and found, amongst other things, that rebounding was helpful in treating both osteo- and rheumatoid arthritis patients. An excellent booklet published by Arthritis Care says

> The right sort of exercise for you will depend on your arthritis, how fit you are, how much exercise you have been used to taking – and what you enjoy. The right sort of exercise cannot harm you, provided you don't push yourself too far or go on too long. The stiff joints which are not exercised become stiffer but for many types of arthritis, gentle, regular exercising is very important.
>
> It's almost the most important way in which you can help yourself. It keeps you mobile, it reduces pain, it

relieves stress (because it is relaxing), and it protects your joints by keeping the muscles strong.

Rebounding gently for two to three minutes a day will reduce pain for many people. We have had people ring us after a week and say, 'My pain has gone.' It strengthens the muscles and generally gets the body healthier in a way that most people with this illness can cope with.

The relief felt by arthritis sufferers is often quite dramatic. People who live in constant pain can reduce it and begin to get more mobile, but it is necessary to use a bouncer properly. Stand relaxed and bounce *very* gently, and watch your barriers (see page 46). DO NOT be tempted to do too much at any one time. A little and often is what works best. If you do get carried away and do too much you will get your pain back. In this event if you do what we describe as the therapeutic rock (see page 52) for a minute two or three times you should find your pain has reduced again.

Rebounding can take the place of jogging and more strenuous and time-consuming exercise. Exercise is necessary to prevent excess calcium loss from the spine and other major bones, and so can bring about wonderful changes in many arthritics.

Asthma

Because rebounding is 68 per cent more oxygen efficient than other exercise – which means it seems easier to do – most people with asthma can do it and, of course, get fitter and feel better. Many have told us that after a few days bouncing they can manage without using their ventilators. The message for any asthma sufferer must be *gently does it,* but it has worked for some.

Back Problems

Rebound exercise is an alternative to jogging which has all the advantages and none of the disadvantages and some advantages of its own. It dissipates the impact stress experienced when running or jumping on a hard surface, and therefore does not place undue strain on the back.

Balance

When jumping or running on a rebounder the surface gives way in all directions and this gives optimum stimulation to the body's balancing mechanisms. It can therefore help to improve balance and co-ordination.

Blood Pressure, Cholesterol and Circulation

The stronger the heart muscles, the less work they have to do to pump the blood around the body. Aerobic exercise, which uses oxygen as its source of energy, makes increased demands on the heart, which causes it to strengthen, thus improving circulation. At the same time the increased lymphatic circulation removes more waste, including cholesterol, from the blood vessels, leaving the way for the blood clearer. This should mean a reduction in blood pressure. It can also help with varicose veins. It has now been medically accepted that exercise reduces the cholesterol level, and we have a number of letters from people who have found that their cholesterol level has gone down following the start of a rebound exercise programme.

Colds and Sore Throats

Rebounding stimulates the lymphatic/immune system, and it has worked for both of us for six years. Neither my husband nor I have had a cold or sore throat in all that time. We have had the start of both, but a few minutes gentle rebounding frequently, perhaps four or five times a day, has seen the back of it. (See therapeutic rock, page 52.)

Diabetes

We have heard of diabetics whose blood sugar level has become stable after a week or two of regular rebounding, although there is no medical evidence for this claim as yet.

Fatigue

Fatigue, or as some doctors call it 'twentieth-century blues', is very common. People cannot be bothered to do things and feel that nothing is worthwhile and life is not worth living. Just make the effort and get on to a rebounder – even in the first few minutes you may find yourself smiling. As your lymph starts to circulate more efficiently you should get back that 'good to be alive' feeling and feel a sense of well-being and energy.

Headaches, Migraine and Stiff Neck

Many people tell us that they used to have headaches and migraine, and that they go away when they start to rebound. This is probably due to the way in which rebounding will relax the body and relieve stress and tension. Many headaches seem to be caused by stress in the muscles at the back of the neck and across the top of the shoulders. Exercise does cause the body to produce greater amounts of serotonin, which is the body's natural way of bringing about a reduction in stress. We have also learned that acupuncturists stimulate the point which governs the lymphatic system when they treat for headaches, and rebounding stimulates the lymphatic circulation.

If you have a headache, rebound gently for a minute or two. If it does not relieve it the first time, try again about an hour later. Generally this also helps a stiff neck.

Health

Dr Gideon, a member of the Olympics Committee, has stated that rebound exercise appears an ideal aerobic exercise activity for all ages, designed to promote and maintain a healthy mind and body. In 1990 some statistics were published by the Sports Council showing that 30 per cent of adults do some vigorous activity, but only six per cent do sufficient for it to have an effect on their health. This means that 94 per cent of the adult population do not take sufficient physical activity to help to maintain a healthy body and, possibly, mind. Increased physical activity can, as you will have read earlier, have a marked effect on how you feel and on your general health. Rebounding affects every cell, muscle, and organ in the body simultaneously, doing all that other forms of aerobic exercise can and more.

Heart Complaints

The British Heart Foundation has said that failing to exercise is as bad for your heart as smoking 20 cigarettes a day. People who have had heart surgery are advised to start a gentle exercise programme as part of the rehabilitation, and many hospitals are using rebounding as part of their rehabilitation programmes after heart surgery.

Hyperactivity

This seems to be a growing problem with children and we wonder if the problem is connected with a lack of physical activity. Many play no games and neither do they have compulsory exercise lessons. We have found that rebounders are very popular with children of all ages. Some who have been a problem to their parents, aggressive and difficult to cope with, have calmed down after a few days' use of a rebounder.

Myalgic Encephalomyelitis (ME)

ME is generally considered to be an immune-deficiency problem and as the immune system is strengthened, following upon improved lymphatic stimulation, this should alleviate ME, and possibly cure it altogether. We know of a number of people who had ME when they started rebounding and have not got it now. There is no proof that rebounding cures ME, but people who have it should start to gain energy and a sense of well-being in the first few days and go on to get fitter and healthier.

Multiple Sclerosis (MS)

Rebounding will not cure MS, but it can help people suffering from it to feel better and get fitter. Many people with debilitating illnesses have told us that bouncing helps them to get a feeling of well-being and energy, and the body gets fitter and stronger so helping to fight the illness.

Osteoporosis

This is a condition which leads to brittle bones and an increased chance of fracture. One woman in four can expect to develop the condition and we believe that one man in ten is likely to suffer from it. As we said earlier, NASA found that a strenuous programme of rebounding/trampolining strengthened the bones of the returning astronauts who had lost bone mass while in space, and exercise is necessary to prevent excess calcium loss from the spine and other major bones. It is lack of exercise, rather than old age (as was once believed) that leads to osteoporosis. It is now generally accepted that a 30-minute walk every day will improve osteoporosis, and five minutes rebounding is approximately equal to a 30-minute walk.

Premenstrual Tension (PMT)

Many have told us that their PMT has improved. If bloated, an extra minute or two bounce the day before is helpful. Regular rebounding will help you have an easier time. If you have a headache, feel tense or bloated, try to fit in several extra bounces the night before. Just a one minute therapeutic rock will help.

Parkinson's Disease

Rebounding will not cure Parkinson's Disease, but it has helped with mobility, balance and general health, and gives a sense of well-being. People have told us that they feel bouncing helps keep the illness at bay.

Skin, Hair and Nails

Dermatitis can improve with this exercise. Your skin is the largest organ and rebounding gives a gentle, all-over massage every time. Hair and nails also improve with fitness.

Sleeping

If you have problems with sleeping you will almost certainly find that one or two minutes therapeutic rock (see page 52) just before you go to bed will be helpful. If you wake in the night and cannot get back to sleep, whether from pain or feeling restless, get up and bounce gently for one or two minutes and you will probably get back to sleep.

Slimming

Rebounding stimulates the metabolic rate. A slim body is a healthy body; it produces less strain on your heart. Many people have lost three to four stone (up to 56 pounds) without dieting, but it is important to bounce frequently. The metabolic rate is speeded up each time you bounce but drops again very quickly, so try to bounce for two to three minutes first thing in the morning and then again 20 to 30 minutes before you eat. This will keep your metabolic rate at a higher level.

It is quite usual for people to lose two or three inches off the waist and hips in the first week or two. This is the body getting fitter and tightening up. In the first couple of weeks Peter, my husband, lost about three inches round the middle but no weight.

Sports Injuries

Without imposing the usual skeletal shock an injured sportsman can get back to a little training earlier, which will not only help when he is fully fit but also increase the rate of healing. Do not, however, exceed your personal limits. Many hospitals use rebounding to treat injuries and many professional sportsmen use rebound training to avoid dropping fitness levels too far.

Stress and Tension

Rebounding is the perfect way to clear stress and tension from the body. Every time you bounce you start with the gentle bounce or, as we have called it, the therapeutic rock (see page 52). This can be done for an odd minute when you are feeling stressed. Once you have cleared your initial stress it is just as if the tension trickles out of your finger tips. Try this and remember that if you could be free of excess tension your health would improve.

Strokes

We have worked with many stroke victims. Because of their condition and lack of movement, all the body's systems slow down, often giving a sense of lethargy and depression. After only a few days of very gentle bouncing they generally get a sense of energy and well-being. Some of those whose speech has been affected find that they start to speak more clearly. One person described to us how her mother's conversation – impaired following a stroke – improved after she started rebounding, which indicated that her thinking had also become clearer.

Varicose Veins

Varicose veins are caused by rubbish in and around them. As your lymphatic system improves and disposes of more of the waste in the body, much of what causes this problem will be removed. It has relieved them for quite a few people, including Peter, my husband.

Strengthening Pelvic Floor Muscles

Twenty per cent of older people lose control of their urinary functions. To combat this when doing the basic bounce, contract the pelvic floor muscles to a count of five and let go gently. Do this two or three times a day as a regular part of your workout and you will soon find a great improvement.

Here are extracts from just two of the many letters we have received:

'We have been rebounding for nearly one year. I have MS and my husband has cancer of the lymph glands. We are both improving so much we can't believe it – it's all thanks to you.'

'I was in so much pain I could hardly walk. Within ten days of starting to rebound the pain was gone.'

Chapter 3

Health Check

Before you start any exercise programme you need to know how fit you are. Firstly it will enable you to establish at what sort of level you will be able to start and secondly it will give you a point with which to compare your progress.

If you are suffering from any complaint in respect of which you are taking or have taken medical advice please make sure from your own medical adviser that gentle exercise will not be harmful. If you are currently taking any medication it would be most ill advised to stop without your doctor's approval, however you feel.

Many doctors feel that it is advisable for everyone over about 40 years of age to have regular health checks – particularly to keep an eye on such things as blood pressure and cholesterol – and if you fall into this age group and have not had a recent check it would be a very good idea to do so before starting on any rebounding programme.

How Fit Are You?

There is no single simple way of telling, but answering the questions opposite will give you some idea.

Answer either 'yes' or 'no' for each question.

1. Do you quickly get out of breath walking up hill or even on the flat?
2. Have you ever had any heart problems?
3. Do you ever have chest pains?
4. Do you have high blood pressure?
5. Do you ever feel faint or dizzy?
6. Are you carrying any injuries?
7. Do you have arthritis or joint pain?
8. Do you suffer from osteoporosis?
9. Are you diabetic, asthmatic or epileptic?
10. Are you extremely overweight?
11. Have you been inactive for more than three months?
12. Have you been a heavy smoker?
13. Are you pregnant?
14. Are you on any medication?
15. Does your family have a history of early death by stroke or heart disease?
16. Do you have any middle-ear (balance) problems?
17. Have you had a recent operation?

If you have answered 'yes' to any of the above questions, gentle rebound exercise would probably be a good way to improve your fitness and health. But you MUST start gently and for VERY short times – say 30 seconds only. If you have answered 'no' to all of these questions, congratulations, but you must still start gently and work round your body's barriers or limits (see page 46).

Chapter 4

Choosing a Rebounder

Rebounders can cost anything between £19 and £150. Some units are made of aluminium with aluminium springs and with daily use these springs can pull through the frame with very dangerous results. Some units have nylon or plastic mats which are too springy and do not give the support to your body that is needed for effective use. To the older and less agile they can in fact be quite dangerous and they do not give the same results.

The best type of unit has a polypropylene mat – one of the strongest materials available – and a high-quality steel frame and steel springs. One make is guaranteed for one year for persons up to 22 stones (308 pounds) but should last a lifetime.

One of the difficulties in choosing a rebounder is that they all look very similar and it is only by standing on them and bouncing that you can tell the difference. Many are not guaranteed at all and the manufacturers recommend that if you are over 13 stones (182 pounds) you do not use them. The difference in the weight they will take is significant in that it does show the comparative strength and the level of support that it will give your body while you are using it.

A rebounder is NOT a trampoline and should not be

springy. It needs a firm, self-centring mat that gives a feeling of security. The mat needs to have the correct tension if you are to gain maximum benefit. Exhaustive research and tests have been carried out by some manufacturers to produce what both they and we believe to be a well-designed, good quality and safe rebounder.

We find that the smaller rebounder, and there are some with a diameter of 36 inches, does not give you a safe, stable feeling nor enough room for your feet when bouncing. The rebounder we use is 40 inches in diameter and stands about nine inches from the floor. It will stand on its side when not in use.

WARNING – Beware of cheap rebounders. They do not give the same results. To rebound safely and effectively you must have a high-quality rebounder. Cheaply designed and manufactured units, although similar in looks, simply do not provide the full benefits that are essential in a rebounding programme. You are best using a rebounder approved by the Aerobic Fitness Teachers Association.

What follows is a specification and description of a good and safe rebounder.

Rebounder Specification

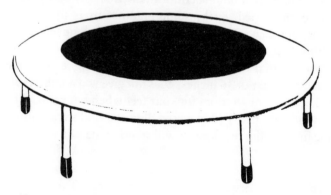

- 18-gauge zinc-plated steel frame with three enamel treatments.

- 7" chrome legs that can be tightened for safety.

- Non-slip heavy-duty rubber feet with reinforced steel washer to take up to 22 stone without 'bottoming out'.

- Specially designed high quality polypropylene weatherproof mat made to an exact specification to ensure an even tension on all 36 reinforced galvanised chrome springs which gives a self-centring bounce. This gives you more confidence and stability.

- Reinforced frame to take the strain of the springs.

- Extra strength stitching to ensure mat does not 'ladder' or 'tear'.

- Washable, aesthetically pleasing covers.

- Spare parts readily available.

- Choice of colour.

- Guarantee (12 months).

The above points are of vital importance in the specification of a rebounder to make it a really good unit and to make it safe. Just as importantly it needs to feel safe and not to give too much bounce.

One thing to watch for is that the legs are attached at the outside edge of the frame, which will mean that the unit is very much less likely to tip if you need to tread on the frame to get onto or off it. This stability is also important when the unit will be used by children, who tend to step onto the edge.

Chapter 5

Exercises and Routines

Owning a rebounder does you no good at all, it's *using* it that makes life better and better. Using it properly makes it work.

Barriers

This section is very important – I suggest that you read it through several times. Each body is different and will react differently to a new form of exercise.

When you first start to bounce stand on the rebounder with feet hip-width apart, knees slightly bent keeping them soft, and relax the whole of your body. Be very aware of your shoulders; many people feel their shoulders going up as they bounce – this is tension – so just give your shoulders a little shake and move them around. By the third time you bounce you should have got rid of that tension.

Think 'bounce', and most people will start to bounce very gently. It seems like magic: as long as you are using a real rebounder it seems to do it for you.

Watch the clock, preferably one with a sweep second hand. Your body will tell you when to stop – make a mental note of the time. You may get a feeling of tension in the calves, in the small of your back, or in the back of your neck, or you could feel dizzy. As soon as you feel one of these things happening, STOP. This is just your body saying, 'I have had enough.' *This is your barrier.* If you had done a minute at this point, the next time you bounce work just under your barrier, say 55 seconds. There is no competition, so if several of you are starting rebounding don't try to do as much as someone else; your body will tell you what is right for you. For best results try to bounce two or three times a day. After a few days try your time again and you will find the time that is good for you.

I cannot emphasize enough that a little and often brings the best results. Use your rebounder when you get out of bed in the mornings; it wakes your system up and speeds up your metabolic rate. If you want to slim, rebound 20 to 30 minutes before eating for whatever time you have decided on. When you come home from business, shopping or doing the garden, it will relax you and then you will feel new energy.

People with arthritis have to take extra care. Many lose their pain in the first week of rebounding, but some will find their pain coming back at some point. If this happens, stop and think:

1. Have I added a new exercise?

2. Am I doing longer?

3. Am I bouncing more energetically?

If so, go back a step and the pain should go.

If you feel a tremendous spurt of energy and do a really hard workout and put yourself in pain, don't panic, just do the basic bounce (therapeutic rock) for one minute a few times and your pain will go.

Always leave a half-hour gap in between using your rebounder. As you rebound all your energies are raised, but they start to drop quite quickly, and if you bounce again before they settle it could make you dizzy.

If you start to tingle, that's fine, that is just your lymphatic system letting you know that it is getting going. You might feel it in your fingers, legs or shoulders, which proves that it does go right round your body almost immediately.

Slowly does it

We suggest that everyone starts gently at 30 seconds a time. The young and healthy will quickly build up to a workout if they want to, but the older or ill will have to take it at a more leisurely pace, adding perhaps 30 seconds a week.

Rebounding is a very potent form of exercise, and for good results from the start it is very important that you build up both the time and the amount of energy used slowly. We cannot stress enough that more does not necessarily mean better and the fact that every body is different. Some people have had wonderful results by rebounding for a very short time but frequently.

Many people start as suggested with 30 seconds to one minute at a time, and then because they feel so good they step up to five, six or even seven minutes, and are surprised that their pain comes back. So if you are at a point where you are bouncing and feeling better, keep at that point for a while, say at least two or three days, before you go on longer or add another exercise to your workout.

Do not push yourself to do too much. If you are doing two minutes at a time and getting good results, don't think 'I ought to be doing more.' Feel your own body. People who are reasonably fit may quickly progress to 5 or even 10 minutes at a time, but some ill people who have used a rebounder for months have had good results with 30 seconds at a time (or less).

Never push through your barrier particularly if you are older or ill in any way.

Remember that you can bounce as many times a day as you like so long as you leave 30 minutes between sessions.

After using a rebounder for six years I feel fit and well and energetic, and when I rebound to music I want to jump and do some of the more energetic exercises and, in fact, I can – but always within two days my arms start to hurt. My arms were and, I suppose, still are my weakest point. I find that as long as I stick to the basic exercises and gentle jogging I feel fine. It is a very old saying that a chain is as strong as its weakest link, and our bodies are the same. Rebounding will affect your weakest point first. When used correctly, bouncing will strengthen the weakest part, but you must listen to what your body tells you. If bouncing starts to hurt, you are doing too much.

Exercise Programme

It is worth deciding in advance just when you are going to rebound. First thing in the morning, within five minutes of getting out of bed, is the very best time. You may think that you cannot face it or that you are in too much of a rush, but you can do two to three minutes while your tea cools, so you will have lost no time at all. You will find that it wakes your body up and makes you feel good and starts your day well.

If you are at home during the day, two to three minutes 20 to 30 minutes before your midday meal and again before your evening meal will be of benefit. If you are working, bounce as soon as you get home and it will relieve the stress and tension of the day and give you fresh energy – the more tired you feel the better the result.

Try your programme every day for the first week and you will know how much good it is doing you. If your body gets into the habit of set times it will be easier to do. Then if you fancy it you can have an odd minute after shopping or too much gardening or just whenever you feel like it.

Once a day will do you good, twice is better, and three times is what gives really wonderful results.

On the following pages there are a number of exercises we have given as suggestions. We advise that you use these to build up a routine from your 30-second or minute start, adding 30 seconds a week. You can choose any exercise you fancy and sort yourself out a routine that you like. Remember that you need to take it gently and build up in easy stages and pay proper regard to your barriers.

The exercises need to start with a warm-up, such as the basic bounce. If you start too energetically you can cause harm to muscles and unnecessary pain. You should not feel any pain at all.

At the end of this chapter is a suggested workout routine. You will notice that the mobilizing exercises come first; this should always be the case as you build up your routine. If any exercise hurts or is unsuitable for you, by all means leave it out, but mobilize as much of your body as possible. If you want to just bounce, that is all right. Remember that all of the exercises are *small, slow* movements.

BASIC POSTURE

- Stand in the centre of the rebounder
- Feet hip-width apart
- Knees slightly bent (soft)
- Relax the shoulders
- Look straight ahead

Try to get the posture right before you continue.

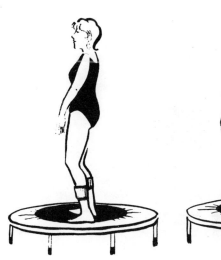
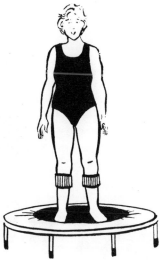

BASIC POSTURE, SIDE   BASIC POSTURE, FRONT

BASIC BOUNCE (THERAPEUTIC ROCK)

- Get into the basic posture
- Very gently flex the knees slightly and think bounce (you will bounce very gently)
- Keep your feet flat on the mat as you bounce
- Keep it gentle

You need to be able to do the basic bounce comfortably for one minute before you add any other exercise to your routine.

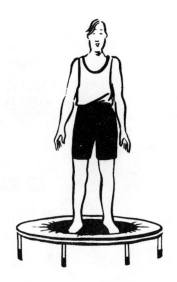

BASIC BOUNCE / THERAPEUTIC ROCK

As time goes by I become more and more interested in this exercise. There is very little movement, just a very gentle rocking motion. Concentrate on your centre of gravity – in your abdomen about three inches below your navel – as you bounce and you will find the results are fantastic.

The therapeutic rock is best used for one minute at a time and will help to clear:

- headaches
- stress and tension
- stiff necks
- frozen shoulders
- colds, sore throats and flu

It is advisable to repeat this every hour or so for a few hours, when you should notice a reduction in the symptoms – possibly they will have gone altogether. Several times at workshops we have found that after three short sessions on the bouncer 'frozen' shoulders have cleared completely. If you have a cold, you will definitely need to repeat this exercise every hour if you want to clear it. It is best to start as soon as you feel the beginning of it – often a prickling feeling at the back of the throat. It does not work every time, but we have found it very successful for us. Neither Peter nor I have had a cold develop since we started rebounding six years ago.

ARM MOBILISER

- Keep doing the basic bounce very gently
- Bend your arms at the elbows with your hands in front of you
- Rotate the hands in one direction and then in the other
- Do this five times with each hand

- With hands in front lift the palms up to the shoulders then relax them in front
- Do this five times with each hand

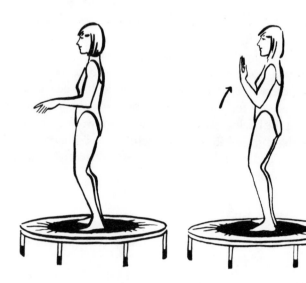

ARM MOBILISER 1   ARM MOBILISER 2

SHOULDER MOBILISER

- Relax your hands at your sides
- Raise one shoulder gently towards the ear, relax down again and do the other side
- Do this five times with each shoulder

- Keep your hands at your sides
- Gently circle your shoulders forwards five times
- Gently circle your shoulders backwards five times
- Do this five times forwards and five times backwards

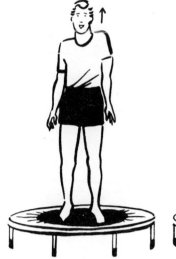 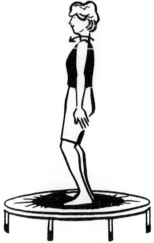

SHOULDER MOBILISER 1   SHOULDER MOBILISER 2

HAND SHAKE

- Relax your hands at your sides
- Whilst still bouncing very gently shake each hand five times

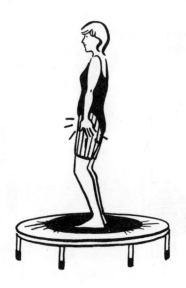

HAND SHAKE

NECK MOBILISER

- Keep doing the basic bounce
- Look to the left
- Look to the front
- Look to the right
- Look to the front
- Do this five times on each side
- Keep the movement small and the head level

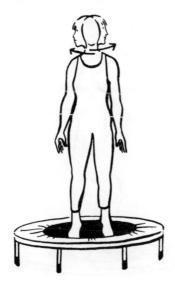

NECK MOBILISER

WALK KNEES

- Assume the basic posture
- Relax
- Very gently walk the knees in a rhythmical motion one after the other
- Make sure your feet stay flat on the mat, not leaving it at all
- Swing your arms gently if you want to, as if you are having a gentle stroll but not going anywhere

Do this exercise very gently for 30 seconds.

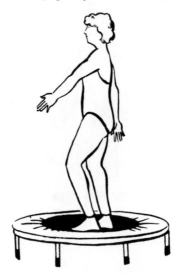

WALK KNEES

PEDAL FEET

- Assume the basic posture
- Relax
- Very gently raise alternate heels in a rhythmical motion, keeping your toes on the mat
- Swing your arms gently if you want to

Do this exercise for 30 seconds.

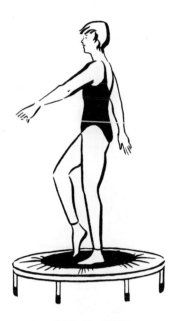

PEDAL FEET

LEG SIDE

- Assume the basic posture
- Relax
- Take your right leg out to the side, touch your foot to the mat
- Return to centre
- Take your left leg out to the side, touch your foot to the mat
- Return to centre
- Alternate from side to side with a gentle bounce in between each movement
- Gently swing your arms in time with your legs if you want to

Do this exercise for 30 seconds.

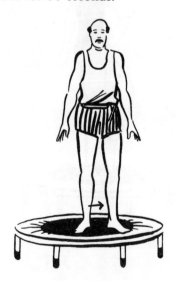

LEG SIDE

LEG FORWARD

- Assume the basic posture
- Relax
- Take your right leg forward, touch your foot to mat
- Return to centre
- Take your left leg forward, touch your foot to mat
- Return to centre
- Alternate gently from foot to foot, with a gentle bounce in between
- Swing your arms gently if you want to

Do this gently for 30 seconds.

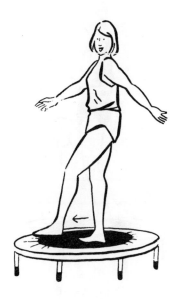

LEG FORWARD

KNEE RAISE

- Assume the basic posture
- Relax
- Lift your right knee in front
- Return to the mat
- Lift your left knee in front
- Return to the mat
- Alternate gently with small lifts
- Gently bounce as you alternate

Do this gently for 30 seconds.

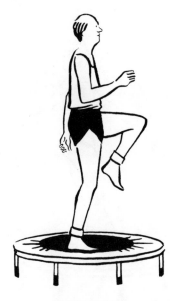

KNEE RAISE

FRONT KICK

- Assume the basic posture
- Relax
- Kick your right foot forward
- Return to mat
- Kick your left foot forward
- Return to the mat
- Alternate from foot to foot
- Gently bounce as you alternate

Do this for 30 seconds.

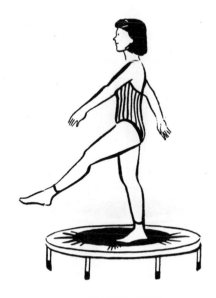

FRONT KICK

SIDE KICK

- Assume the basic posture
- Relax
- Kick your right foot out to the side
- Return to the mat
- Kick your left foot out to the side
- Return to the mat
- Alternate from foot to foot
- Gently bounce as you alternate

Do this for 30 seconds.

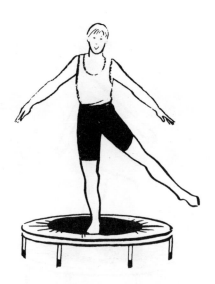

SIDE KICK

SMALL TWIST

- Assume the basic posture
- Keeping your toes on the mat –
- Bounce the heels to the right
- Bounce the heels to the centre
- Bounce the heels to the left
- Bounce the heels to the centre
- Start again
- Swing your arms gently in time with your feet

Do this for 30 seconds.

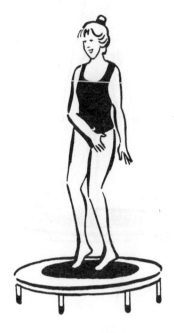

SMALL TWIST

GENTLE HOPSCOTCH

- Assume the basic posture, but with feet further apart
- Take your right foot behind
- Return to centre
- Take your left foot behind
- Return to centre
- Bounce gently as you alternate

Do this for 30 seconds.

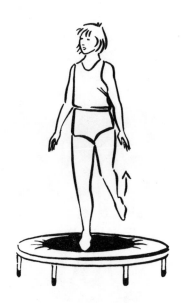

GENTLE HOPSCOTCH

SIDE-TO-SIDE ROCK

- Assume the basic posture, but with feet further apart
- Keep feet flat on the rebounder
- Bounce to the right very gently
- Bounce to the left very gently
- Try to double bounce on either side, alternating gently

Do this for 30 seconds.

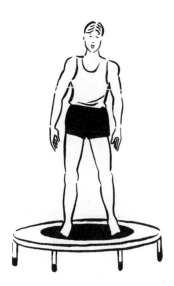

SIDE-TO-SIDE ROCK

Any exercise you try should be done on a low level, bouncing very gently and not bouncing off the mat. You should exercise around your barriers, as explained at the beginning of this chapter, starting gently with a one-minute basic bounce and gradually adding on 30 seconds as and when you feel capable. REMEMBER: IF ANYTHING HURTS OR YOU DO NOT LIKE A PARTICULAR EXERCISE, STOP, OR DO A DIFFERENT EXERCISE.

Below we have laid out a workout suggestion that may suit you. Remember that you add only 30 seconds on each week or when you are feeling up to it.

If you have any debilitating condition it will take you a long while to work up to anything like five and a half minutes. It could take months, or you may never get there. The object is to feel better, so do only what suits you.

WORKOUT SUGGESTION

Basic Bounce	1 minute
Arm Mobiliser	30 seconds
Shoulder Mobiliser	30 seconds
Neck Mobiliser	30 seconds
Walk Knees	30 seconds
Pedal Feet	30 seconds
Knee Raise	30 seconds
Front Kick	30 seconds
Basic Bounce	1 minute

Remember this is a suggestion, have fun and experiment.

If at any point you wish to progress much beyond five and a half minutes you must incorporate stretching into your routine. We have given you some ideas for this in the next chapter.

Chapter 6

Further Rebound Exercises

Rebounding must be the easiest and most convenient way of keeping fit. You can do a 30-minute workout at home three or four times a week at a time to suit yourself and at your own level, which will give you all the physical benefits of a regular workout without either the skeletal shock or the inconvenience of having to go somewhere else at a certain time. Although elsewhere we recommend bare feet, if you are doing a workout and rebounding for more than 10 minutes it is advisable to wear training shoes.

It is important if using your rebounder as a part of your fitness programme that you do an appropriate warm-up, and incorporate a stretching routine. You should stretch the major muscle groups after they have been warmed up, and before you begin your aerobic training. It is also important to stretch at the end of your routine, to prevent muscle soreness.

Below are a few stretches we recommend, but they are by no means all the stretches you can do.

HAMSTRING STRETCH

- Place one foot on the rebounder, the other on the floor (feet should be pointed in the same direction)
- Push down the heel that is on the floor
- The back leg should be straight
- The front leg is bent
- Push forward gently and hold for 10 seconds
- Do both sides

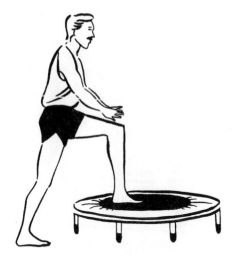

HAMSTRING STRETCH

CALF STRETCH

- Keep the same position as in the last exercise
- Straighten the front leg
- Bend the back leg
- Reach for the toe of the front leg
- Hold the stretch for 10 seconds
- Do both sides

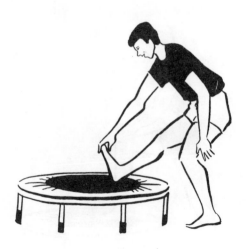

CALF STRETCH

QUAD STRETCH

- Place the rebounder on its side (it will support itself)
- Hold the edge of the rebounder
- Lift your right heel towards your bottom, your knee pointing at the floor
- Keep your left leg slightly bent
- Hold for 10 seconds
- Do both sides

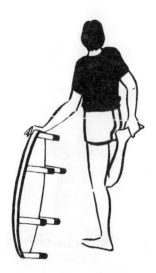

QUAD STRETCH

SHOULDER AND UPPER BACK STRETCH

- Stand with your feet shoulder-width apart
- Bend your knees slightly
- Tighten your bottom
- Raise both arms above your head
- Arms straight, palms facing upwards
- Hold stretch for about 10 seconds

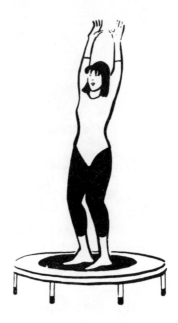

SHOULDER AND UPPER BACK STRETCH

The following three exercises are specific training exercises for the fit and are just a sample of what can be done.

JOGGING EXERCISE

- Stand in the centre of the rebounder
- Gently start to jog, raising one foot after the other
- Land on flat feet not on your toes
- If you want to work harder raise your knees higher
- Add arm movements in time with your legs

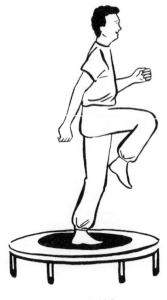

JOGGING

Skiing

Rebounding is an excellent way of getting legs in trim for
skiing holidays. Some users have found that it effectively
extends their holiday by three days or so, the time that they
have previously had to use to prepare the muscles for skiing
for longer periods, and they have not had the usual aches
and stiffness. Here are a couple of exercises specially for
pre-ski training. You should incorporate them into a routine
that includes a warm-up and stretching.

SLALOM

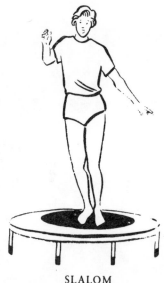

- Keep feet and knees very
  close together
- Bounce to the left and
  then to the right
- Keep the knees bent as you
  bounce from side to side
- You can incorporate
  45-degree turns as you
  bounce if you want to
  make it harder

SLALOM

DOWNHILL

- Place feet roughly hip-width apart
- Keep feet flat on the mat
- Bend your knees so that the thighs and calves are at right angles
- Pretend that you are heading down a ski slope
- Bounce the feet up and down as if absorbing the bumps
- Start slowly and build up gradually

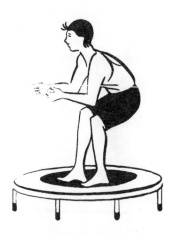

DOWNHILL

Rebounding can be used to maintain a higher level of fitness for any sport. Even while you are suffering from a sports injury you can still exercise without causing any aggravation to the injury, which helps you maintain your fitness level.

The Rebounder Centre has available a book called *Rebound Aerobics,* which gives aerobic routines specially designed for use on the rebounder. It also shows you how you can use your rebounder for specific area exercises and body toning. For further information see page 96.

Chapter 7

For Those
With Special Needs

If a disability prevents you from rebounding, the same effect
can be achieved if you sit in a chair or wheelchair with your
feet on the mat and let someone else do the bouncing. The
effect transmits through your body and will stimulate the
lymphatic system. This is clearly very useful for the severely
disabled and has had quite remarkable results.

We heard about one woman, aged 83, who was
bedridden for most of the time. She was persuaded to sit
with her feet on the rebounder while her husband bounced.
They did this several times a day and four days later she was
up and doing a little around the kitchen, and rebounding
herself. Eight days after starting she was working in the
kitchen, joking with her husband and enjoying life again.

To our certain knowledge a number of people have found
benefit from this sitting method, and we used it ourselves
after I had an accident and badly damaged my back. It kept
my arthritis at bay for a few days until I could walk again
and seemed to help in coping with the pain of the injury
and its healing. After a few days I was able to bounce for
myself.

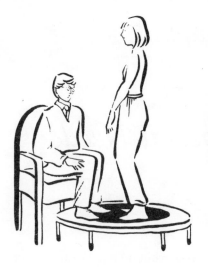

CHAIR

We have heard of other wonderful results. Recently a lady who had been wheelchair-bound for three years was persuaded to sit with her feet on the mat while her daughter bounced. After five weeks she was not only walking but going up and down stairs.

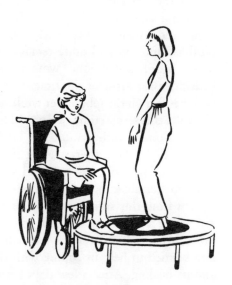

WHEELCHAIR

Support Bars

Support bars that fix onto the rebounder are available. When using a support bar use it gently; it is only to give balance or location. It is important that you remain as relaxed as possible; we find that some people tend to grip the support bar very hard and cause tension unnecessarily. I know that it is not easy to have a light hold on the support bar when you cannot balance, but the bouncer is firm and is not going to spring you into the air (provided that you have the right one). You can take your time to find a position where you will feel happy. Do not ever try to force yourself to do more than is comfortable. A small amount each day can work wonders.

The support bar is a real point of reference for those with visual difficulties. We have seen blind people doing real

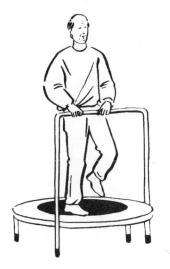

USING THE SUPPORT BAR

aerobic workouts when in the past any exercise except walking had been very difficult for them. And, of course, they can do this in their own home.

At one day centre a young man who had never walked was started off sitting with his feet on a rebounder. He then progressed to standing, with staff to support him and another to bounce him. Then he managed to stand *and bounce himself.* He also sat on the mat and raised himself up and down with the bar. This man is now walking. It took a long time, but it has given him a new life.

Chapter 8

Your Questions Answered

People often have questions about rebounding. Below are those that we are asked most frequently and the answers that we give. Most of these questions are answered in more detail in the relevant chapters of this book.

Q. My friends have been rebounding for about a year now and, as well as many other benefits they have gained, they insist that rebounding can get rid of colds, sore throats and even flu. Can this possibly be true?

A.   Yes, nearly always. Amazing though it may seem, at the first signs of symptoms of a cold (that tickling in the back of the throat) you very gently bounce for a couple of minutes and, if you do this frequently, every hour, you will find that the stimulation of the immune system will effectively wash the germs away.

Q.   Is it good for slimming?

A.   Yes – used correctly. Many people have lost up to two, three or even four stones (56 pounds) without a change of diet. If you rebound in conjunction with a diet that has worked for you before, you should find that your weight loss will be two to three times as quick. Rebounding also helps to keep your energy level up, so that you do not have that listless feeling when you start to reduce your food intake.

Q. Does everybody lose weight from rebounding?

A. No. You will only lose weight if you are carrying surplus. If you are underweight you may well find that you will gain a little as you get fitter.

Q. I rebound twice a day for five minutes 20 to 30 minutes before eating and I have not lost any weight. Why?

A. The lady that asked us this was active and reasonably fit. We suggested that she exercised a little more strenuously and made a particular point that the best time to rebound is within three to five minutes of getting out of bed. Two weeks later she told us that she had lost 7 lbs. 'It just seemed to disappear.' She had not been working up to her barrier. Several people have told us that they bounced for a week or two and did not immediately lose weight, but then it suddenly just dissolved away.

Q. Does it tighten your body?

A. Yes, you will find that your muscle tone improves and with it your shape.

Q. Does rebounding help constipation?

A. Yes – in fact just occasionally we come across someone who gets diarrhoea for the first two or three days after starting to bounce. This is your body getting rid of stored toxins.

Q. Does it help older people?

A. Yes. Rebounding is probably the easiest form of exercise that has ever been invented. There is no skeletal shock and it is 68 per cent more oxygen efficient than any other form of exercise. As you get older your joints tend to stiffen up and your heart and lungs do not work as efficiently as in younger days. It becomes more important to gain the maximum benefit from the energy that you put into exercising, and rebounding is probably the only exercise where you can get more benefit out of it than you put in. Even at an advanced age you can still bounce gently up and down, which you should do without becoming breathless. Several people over 90 years of age are using rebounders regularly and many have said that they feel it has given them a new lease of life.

Q. I have rheumatoid arthritis and found that within a few days of using the rebounder my pain eased and I started to feel better than I had in years. I got to five minutes three times a day and felt very well for 18 months. Now suddenly my pain has increased and I feel as if the rebounder is making it worse. Can that be the case?

A. Yes. If you have gone over your barrier – done too long or bounced too strenuously – it can give you pain. If you are doing the correct amount for your body's condition your pain should decrease. Remember also that rebounding does not *cure* the rheumatoid arthritis. This is a disease that can fluctuate – you have your good patches and your bad ones – and it could be that you are having a bad one and that the five minutes is far too much. Go back to doing one or two minutes at a time for a few days. You will gradually build up your time again.

Q. My mother is in a wheelchair with arthritis. How can she use a rebounder?

A. When someone is wheelchair-bound or bedridden or badly disabled they can sit at the side of the rebounder and put their feet on the mat while someone else bounces gently.

The effect will be transferred through the body of the sitting person and they will quickly feel some reaction. If they are badly disabled and consequently have not exercised for some years they will often feel sensation in parts of the body where there has been none for some time.

Q. My son is handicapped. Will it help him?

A. Many schools and centres for the disabled are now using rebounders and find that it improves general health and fitness, and helps balance and clearer thinking.

Q. My husband did one minute night and morning and it has hurt his legs.

A. We asked what exactly he had done. He had jumped as high as he could stiff legged. Everyone should start with a gentle bounce. Stand straight but relaxed, knees soft, feet flat. Do not go up on your toes – if you want more bounce press down with your heels. This warms up the body for more strenuous exercise, if that is what you want to do. Everyone should start with a gentle warming-up exercise.

Q. How often should I use it?

A. Two or three minutes, two or three times a day seems to work wonders. Many people tell us that they often pop on for a minute because it makes them feel good. You can use it as often as you like *provided* that you leave 30 minutes in between sessions.

Q. Why did I feel dizzy the first time I went on a rebounder?

A. Every body has its own barrier, or limit. If you time yourself on the rebounder and find that you go dizzy at two minutes, that means you have done too much for the time being. You will gradually push back the barrier and be able to go on to two minutes and beyond.

Q. I have heard that rebounding is good for relieving tiredness. Is this so?

A.   Yes – amazing though it may seem, the more tired you feel the more effect it will have. If you bounce after getting home from business, shopping or gardening you will find that the tensions will drop away and that the gentle exercise will create energy and make you feel better right away. Your strain, aches and pains will disappear.

Q. I am sure that my eyesight has improved since I started rebounding. Is that possible?

A.   Yes. As you rebound you unwittingly exercise the eye muscles. Rebounding also relieves stress and tension, and eyesight can improve when stress and tension are reduced. For some people it happens more quickly than for others.

Q. Is rebounding good for headaches or migraine?

A.   Many people have told us that they used to have migraine before they started bouncing, and that they now get them less or not at all.

Q. Is rebounding safe for children?

A.   Children adore it. For them it is probably even more important to have a good, safe rebounder that will not tip and is not too bouncy. Children instinctively know how much they can do and will stop at the right time. If you teach your children a routine upon which they can build you will probably have created a good habit for life, which could make a great difference to their health, strength and well-being. Many parents of hyperactive children have told us that their offspring have calmed down and lost the aggressive attitude within three or four days of a rebounder going into the house.

Q. What is the difference between a rebounder and a trampoline?

A. A trampoline is designed for tricks and acrobatics – without special training it can be very dangerous. A rebounder is an exercise unit designed for exercise of a less strenuous or dangerous nature. Beware of items that look like rebounders but are really little trampolines.

Q. Will the legs come off the rebounder so that I can keep it under the bed?

A. Yes – the legs screw off quite easily, but if you intend to do that each time you use it we would recommend that you do not have one. The best results come from using it for two or three minutes, two or three times a day. You need to be able to get on it at any time.

Q. How heavy is a rebounder? I have arthritis – would I be able to move it?

A. The rebounder weighs 8.5 kgs (just under 19 lbs). The easiest way to move it is to tip it onto its side and roll it like a hoop. The best thing is to leave it down, if possible, but otherwise to put it where you can stand it on its side and put it down easily.

Q. Can a rebounder tip up?

A. It is *very* important to have a good rebounder. The one we recommend will not tip up. We have had a heavy man jump on the edge without it tipping. Because it has six legs set on the extreme outside of the steel frame, it is almost impossible to tip it up accidentally. Some of the cheaper ones are not so stable and will tip comparatively easily.

Q. Are they very bouncy? I am in my sixties and have heard how good rebounding is for older people, but I feel very nervous about bouncing up in the air.

A. The rebounder we use has a firm, self-centring mat. When you first stand on it it feels almost solid. Cheaper rebounders have mats that are much more bouncy, and you might fall off.

Q. *Is the effect purely psychological?*

A. If you feel better, does it matter? So far as we can see there is some psychological benefit, but there are many physiological reasons why people feel better. Research at Purdue University in the USA on 60 middle-aged people in sedentary jobs found that their emotional stability, self-sufficiency and confidence improved after they started a physical exercise programme.

Chapter 9

Bouncing Miracles: A Few Personal Stories

In this chapter we include extracts from some of the letters we have received from people who have started rebounding to combat the symptoms of various illnesses and conditions.

'My husband has Parkinson's disease and was shuffling along. After using the bouncer for a month he now walks very much better and can climb stairs – he hasn't been able to do this for two years. Our doctor says it won't cure him but it will certainly benefit him.'

'After 16 years of suffering with arthritis in the spine and hips I have found much relief after using the rebounder for just one month.'

'Just a few lines to say how very pleased I am with the results of the rebounder . . . I suffer from severe osteo-arthritis and angina and to date have had two heart attacks. Consequently I became quite debilitated, no energy, no enthusiasm, no anything really . . . All that has changed.

My general health and sense of well-being has improved enormously and my appetite has returned and I am now quite energetic.'

'I used to attend a keep-fit class once a week in order to have some exercise amidst a very busy life in which I have a demanding full-time job and a home and family. The regular exercise every day has been most beneficial and my outlook is now much calmer.'

'As I am almost 69 years old I don't go in for anything very acrobatic but starting with very gentle bouncing I can now easy-jog for some minutes without discomfort to feet, knees or hips. Afterwards I feel marvellous!! And it lasts! Since starting this exercise I can feel the positive benefit to lungs, heart and circulation. My whole outlook is happier. I am more energetic generally, also I seem to be sleeping better.'

'I have lost one stone (14 pounds) in three months (from 12½ stone to 11½ stone) and my body muscles are all tight and firm. I have lost my sagging belly and two chins and look and feel like a commando ready for a campaign . . . Thanks to my rebounder I am fitter and more mentally agile than I was at 30 even though I am now 50.'

'I have got MS. I did notice a difference straight away. I no longer needed a painkiller before I went to bed . . . plus I sleep so much better. I find my legs are becoming stronger. Two days after starting rebounding I walked to the top of the garden. I had not been there for a good six months . . . Rebounding has lifted my spirits.'

'I am about 81 years old and following a severe illness I wasn't able to walk very far and so I have had very little exercise. I started on my rebounder very gently and am now up to three minutes three times a day and I am feeling much better already.'

'All my life I have had trouble in getting out of bed and getting going. Before it has been 9 o'clock in the office and about 10 o'clock before I really got going. Now I get up at 7 o'clock and get on my rebounder. After five minutes I am ready to go. I get in the office at 8 o'clock and work! That gives me nearly two extra hours a day – 10 hours a week. A whole working day more – and I feel great!'

'I was born 35 years ago with a congenital hip dislocation although it wasn't discovered until I was about four years old by which time the damage had been done. I have spent much of my life in hospital having numerous operations and treatment . . . Some four to five months ago I discovered your course on rebounding. I was amazed at how quickly I felt the benefits. My mobility has been greatly improved. I can bend far more easily and have far less pain.'

'Varicose veins have disappeared in one leg and almost gone in the other.'

'My husband has had a dry scaly skin all his life. Tried many remedies and seen specialists with little result. Since rebounding his skin is smooth with no sign of scaling.'

'After purchasing a rebounder my arthritis is not so painful, my blood pressure has gone down, my weight has gone from 11st 8lbs to 10st 12lbs. I am more than pleased.'

Chapter 10

Summary of Key Points

Finally here are a few reminders to summarise the things that we have found to be important.

1. If you have not been exercising regularly start gently and for a very short period of time – I suggest 30 seconds.

2. Remember your personal barriers or limitations. If anything hurts or feels uncomfortable, STOP.

3. Do not try to progress too quickly.

4. Do not worry how long it takes you to extend the time of your exercise sessions as long as you feel better in the meantime.

5. We do not claim that rebounding *cures* anything, but that it helps people to get fitter in a way they can manage and that makes it easier to cope with the symptoms of most illnesses, especially pain, which is usually reduced in a few days.

6. If it starts to hurt when it was not before you could be going through a bad patch – step your rebounding back a bit and do not be too energetic.

7. Keep in mind that the object is to feel better, not to compete with anyone else.

DO
- Stand relaxed
- Keep your knees soft
- Feel your body
- Be aware of your barrier time
- Remember that a little and often works wonders
- Stand flat footed – if you want more height on your bounce press down with your heels
- Build up the time you bounce slowly
- Remember that more is not necessarily better

DON'T
- Stand stiff and/or tense
- Have your knees stiff and/or braced
- Go up on your toes
- Push through your barrier
- Jump off the rebounder
- Jump high in the air

Further Reading

Alternative Medicine, Readers Digest, London.

Arthritis Care, published by Arthritis Care, 18 Stephenson Way, London NW1 2HD and obtainable by sending stamped and self-addressed envelope size at least 9"×6".

Barnard, Christian, *The Body Machine,* Hamlyn, London.

Carter, Albert, *The Miracles of Rebounding,* available from M. & P. Hawkins, The Rebounder Centre, Leicester, UK.

Conley, Rosemary, *Metabolism Booster Diet,* Arrow Books, London.

Egli, Markus, *Rebound Training,* available from M. & P. Hawkins, The Rebounder Centre, Leicester, UK.

Fisk, James, *Your Painful Neck and Back,* Arrow Books, London.

The Health of The Nation, H.M.S.O.

Kenton, Leslie, *Ultrahealth,* Ebury Press, London.

Leaf, Alexander, *Youth in Old Age,* McGraw & Hill, Maidenhead.

Rose, Colin, *The Mind and Body Diet,* Accelerated Learning Systems.

Wynn-Williams, Sue, 'The PT Bouncer', *Physiotherapy Journal,* Vol. 70, no. 3, March 1984.

THE REBOUNDER CENTRE
51/53 Nevanthon Road, Leicester LE3 6DR
Phone 0116 285 8929

The Rebounder Centre is the first centre of its kind in the U.K. – probably in the world. It is a place where anyone and everyone is welcome to come in and have a go on a professional rebounder. You can learn how to use one to suit your body whatever your present state of health. There is no charge and you do not need to book.

ALSO
at the centre we give
talks and demonstrations.
Workshops are held regularly.
Please contact the Centre for details.
Send for a FREE information pack.

A GOOD QUALITY REBOUNDER IS ESSENTIAL.
WARNING – BEWARE OF CHEAP IMITATIONS
They do not give the same results.
Be careful – it is your body you are risking.